Lung Cancer

The Guide for Surviving and Building Resilience While Living with or Preventing Incurable Lung Cancer

Regina Williams

Copyright © 2020 Regina Williams

All rights reserved. No part of this publication may be reproduced, distributed, or transmitted in any form or by any means, including photocopying, recording, or other electronic or mechanical methods, without the prior written permission of the publisher, except in the case of brief quotations embodied in critical reviews and specific other non-commercial uses permitted by copyright law.

ISBN: 978-1-63750-246-4

Table of Contents

LUNG CANCER 1

INTRODUCTION 5

CHAPTER 1 7
- TREATING OF LUNG CANCER? 7
- HOW EXPERTS DIAGNOSE LUNG MALIGNANCY? 7
  - *How Doctors Determine Lung Malignancy Stages?* 19
  - *What is the Procedure for Lung Cancers?* 21

CHAPTER 2 38
- CAUSES OF LUNG CANCER 38
- HOW SMOKING CAUSES LUNG CANCER 38
- TYPES OF LUNG CANCER 39
  - *Risk factors* 40
  - *Prevention of Lung Cancer* 43

CHAPTER 3 47
- SYMPTOMS OF LUNG CANCER 47
- DIAGNOSIS 48
- STAGING OF CANCER 51
  - *Treatment* 53

CHAPTER 4 56
- PHASES OF LUNG CANCER 56
- RISK FACTORS FOR LUNG CANCER 59
- LUNG CANCERS AND SMOKING 62
- FACTS AND FIGURES ABOUT LUNG CANCER 63

CHAPTER 5 66
- WHAT ARE PULMONARY NODULES? 66
- HOW COMMON ARE PULMONARY NODULES? 66
- WHAT CAN CAUSE PULMONARY NODULES? 67
- WHAT ARE THE SYMPTOMS OF PULMONARY NODULES? 69

    How is Pulmonary nodules Diagnosed? 70

    How are Pulmonary nodules Treated? 74

CHAPTER 6 77

    LUNG NODULES AND BENIGN LUNG TUMOUR 77

    WHAT ARE THE SYMPTOMS OF BENIGN LUNG NODULES AND TUMOURS? 78

    HOW ARE BENIGN LUNG NODULES AND TUMOURS DIAGNOSED? 81

        Treatment of Benign Lung Nodules and Tumours 83

CHAPTER 7 85

    WHAT'S METASTATIC LUNG MALIGNANCY? 85

    HOW DOES METASTATIC LUNG CANCERS DEVELOP? 87

    HOW IS METASTATIC LUNG MALIGNANCY DIAGNOSED? 88

        How is metastatic lung tumour treated? 89

        How can metastatic lung tumour be prevented? 91

CHAPTER 8 93

    WHEN LUNG MALIGNANCY SPREADS TO THE BRAIN 93

    SYMPTOMS OF LUNG TUMOUR WITH BRAIN METASTASES 94

    SYMPTOMS 95

        Diagnosis 97

        Treatment 99

        Brain-Metastasis Specific Treatments 103

Introduction

This guide for surviving and building resilience while living with or preventing incurable lung cancer is an important book for all cancer, as it has uncovered the holy grail those who want to optimize their chances for cure have been seeking.

Lung tumour causes mutations in cells. Typically, your body programs cells to die at a particular stage in their life cycle to avoid overgrowth. Malignancy overrides this training, leading to cells overdevelopment and multiplying when they shouldn't; the growth of cells leads to the introduction of tumours and the harmful effects of cancer.

In lung cancer, this design of cell overgrowth occurs in the lungs (essential organs for breathing and gas exchange); doctors typically diagnose two lung cancer types, small cell, and non-small cell, depending on how they appear under a microscope. One is much more likely to have non-small cell lung malignancy than a low cell.

However, anyone taking tobacco and constant contact

with smoke can boost the likelihood of developing lungs tumour. Lungs cancer can also be improved if one has a brief history of contact with inhaled chemicals or other poisons; even if this contact with chemicals and other toxins was in the past, it might cause changes in lung cells that lead to tumour.

This book will walk you through what to do to avoid lung cancer and also what to do to get better if you have lung cancer. It is filled with important information for everyone, whether struggling with cancer or not.

Chapter 1

Treating of Lung Cancer?

The treating of lung cancer takes a team approach. *Medical oncologists* are cosmetic surgeons specialized in removing malignancies, *Thoracic doctors* or *general cosmetic surgeons* could also surgically treat lung malignancies, *Medical and rays' oncologists* are specialists in the treating of malignancies with medications and rays' therapy, respectively; other specialists who may be engaged in the treatment of individuals with lung cancers include *pain and palliative treatment specialists*, as well as pulmonary specialists (medical pulmonologists).

How Experts Diagnose Lung Malignancy?

Doctors use an array of diagnostic methods and assessments to diagnose lung tumour. These include the next:

- *The annals and physical examination* may reveal the existence of symptoms or signs that are suspicious for lung cancer. Furthermore, to requesting about symptoms and risk factors for cancer development such as smoking, doctors may identify signs of inhaling and exhaling difficulties, airway blockage, or attacks in the lungs. Cyanosis, a bluish colour of your skin and the mucous membranes credited to insufficient air in the bloodstream, suggests jeopardized function credited to chronic disease of the lung. Similarly, changes in the cells of the toenail mattresses, known as *clubbing*, also may indicate chronic lung disease.

- *The chest X-ray* is the most typical diagnostic step that exposes any new symptoms of lung cancer. The upper body X-ray process often requires a view from the trunk to leading of the upper body and a view from the medial side. Like any X-ray treatment, upper body X-rays expose the individual briefly to a little number of rays. High body X-rays may reveal dubious areas in the lungs but cannot see whether these areas are cancerous.

Accurately, doctors may identify calcified nodules in the lungs or harmless tumours called *hamartomas* on the upper body X-ray, and this mimic lung malignancy.

- *CT (computerized tomography) scans* may be performed on the upper body, stomach, and brain to examine for both metastatic and lung tumours. CT scans are X-ray techniques that combine multiple images using a computer to create cross-sectional views of your body. A big doughnut-shaped X-ray machine exposes models at different perspectives around your body.

One benefit of CT scans is that they are more delicate than standard upper body X-rays in recognition of lung nodules, i.e., they'll demonstrate more nodules, sometimes doctors give intravenous comparison material before the scan to help delineate the organs and their positions.

The most common side effect can be an adverse reaction to intravenous comparison material given before the procedure. This might result in scratching, an allergy, or hives that generally vanish in short order. Severe anaphylactic reactions (life-threatening allergies with breathing troubles) to the comparison material are uncommon. CT scans of the belly may identify metastatic tumour in the liver organ or adrenal glands, and your physician may order CT scans of the top to reveal the existence and degree of metastatic cancers in the brain.

- The USPSTF recommends a method called a *low-dose helical CT* to check out (or spiral CT check) annually, in current and past smokers between age groups 55 and 80 with at least a 30 pack-year background of using tobacco who've smoked cigarettes within days gone by 15 years. The lung malignancy screening technique seems to increase the probability of recognition of smaller, previously, and curable lung malignancies. Three years of low-dose CT scanning in this group reduced the chance of lung tumour loss of life by 20%. Usage of models and guidelines for examining the results of the tests are reducing the necessity for biopsy to judge recognized nodules; when it is likely high the nodule is not cancerous.

- *Magnetic resonance imaging (MRI) scans* may be appropriate when exact detail in regards to a tumour's location is necessary. The MRI technique uses magnetism, radio waves, and a PC to create images of body constructions. Much like CT scanning, the individual is placed on the moveable bed that is put into the MRI scanning device. You will find no known part effects of MRI scanning, and there is no exposure to rays. The image and quality made by MRI is quite comprehensive and can identify small changes of buildings in the body. People with centre pacemakers, metallic implants, heart valves, and other surgically implanted constructions can't be scanned with an MRI because of the chance that the magnet may move the steel elements of these structures.

- *Positron emission tomography (Family pet) scanning* is a specialized imaging technique that uses short-lived radioactive drugs to create three-dimensional coloured images of these drugs in the tissue in the body. While CT scans and MRI scans take a look at anatomical buildings, Family pet scans measure metabolic activity and the function of cells. Family pet scans can determine whether a tumour cell is positively growing and can certainly help in determining the kind of cells within a specific tumour. In Family pet checking, the patient gets a brief half-lived radioactive medication, receiving approximately the quantity of ray's publicity as two upper body X-rays. The drug accumulates using tissue more than others, concerning the drug that is injected. The medication discharges contaminants known as positrons from whatever cells take them up. As the positrons encounter electrons in the body, a response producing gamma rays occurs — a scanning device information of these gamma rays and maps the region where the radioactive medication has accumulated. *For instance, combining blood sugar (a common power source in the torso) with radioactive material will show where blood sugar is rapidly being utilized, for example, in an ever-growing tumour.* PET checking can also be integrated with CT checking in a method known as PET-CT checking. Integrated PET-CT has been proven to enhance the precision of staging (see below) over Family PET scanning alone.

Bone scans are accustomed to creating images of bone fragments on a screen or film. Doctors may order a bone scan to determine whether a lung malignancy has metastasized to the bone fragments; in the bone check, a little amount of radioactive materials is injected into the bloodstream and gathers in the bone fragments, especially in irregular areas such as those included by metastatic tumours. The radioactive materials are detected with a scanning device, and the image of the bone fragments is documented on a particular film for long term viewing.

- **Sputum cytology**: The medical diagnosis of lung tumour always requires verification of malignant cells with a pathologist, even though symptoms and X-ray studies are suspicious for lung cancers. The simplest solution to set up the analysis is the *study of sputum under a microscope.*

If a tumour is located and has invaded the airways, this process is known as *a sputum cytology exam*, may allow visualization of tumour cells for analysis. It is the most risk-free and inexpensive tissue diagnostic method, but its value is bound since tumour cells won't always be within sputum even if a malignancy exists. Also, non-cancerous cells may sometimes go through changes in a reaction to swelling or injury, which makes them appear to be cancer cells.

- ***Bronchoscopy***: Study of the airways by bronchoscopy *(visualizing the airways through a thin, fiberoptic probe inserted through the nasal area or mouth area)* may reveal regions of tumour that may be sampled *(biopsied)* for medical diagnosis with a pathologist. A tumour in the central regions of the lung or due to the more significant airways is obtainable to sampling using this system. Bronchoscopy may be performed in a same-day outpatient bronchoscopy collection, a working room, or on the hospital ward. The task can be unpleasant, and it needs sedation or anesthesia. While bronchoscopy is relatively safe, it must be completed with a lung specialist *(pulmonologist or doctor),* experienced in the task. Whenever a tumour is visualized and properly sampled, a precise cancer analysis usually can be done. Some patients may cough up dark-brown bloodstream two times after the process. Much more serious but uncommon complications add a higher amount of blood loss, decreased degrees of air in the bloodstream, and centre arrhythmias as well as problems from sedative medications and anesthesia.

- *Needle biopsy*: Fine-needle aspiration (FNA) through your skin, mostly performed with radiological imaging for assistance, may be useful in retrieving cells for medical diagnosis from tumour nodules in the lungs. Needle biopsies are especially helpful when the lung tumour is peripherally situated in the lung rather than accessible to sampling by bronchoscopy.

Doctors administer a little amount of local anesthetic previous to insertion of the slim needle through the upper body wall into the important area in the lung. Cells are suctioned into the syringe and are analysed under the microscope for tumour cells; this process usually is accurate when the cells from the affected area are adequately sampled, however, in some instances, adjacent or uninvolved regions of the lung may be mistakenly tested. A little risk (3%-5%) of the air drip from the lungs (called a pneumothorax, which can be treated) accompanies the task.

- *Thoracentesis*: Sometimes lung malignancies involve the liner tissues of the lungs (pleura), and business leaders to a build-up of liquid in the area between your lungs and upper body wall structure (called a pleural effusion). Aspiration of an example of this liquid with a slim needle (thoracentesis) may reveal the malignancy cells and create the diagnosis. Much like the needle biopsy, a little threat of a pneumothorax is associated with this process.

- *Major surgical treatments*: If none of these methods yields a diagnosis, employ medical solutions to obtain tumor tissue for diagnosis; these range from mediastinoscopy *(analyzing the upper body cavity between your lungs through a surgically placed probe with biopsy of tumor people or lymph nodes that may contain metastases)* or thoracotomy *(operative starting of the upper body wall structure for removal or biopsy of the tumor)*. Having a thoracotomy, ultimately removal of lung malignancy is uncommon, and both mediastinoscopy and thoracotomy bring the dangers of major surgical treatments (problems such as blood loss, infection, and risks from anesthesia and medications). Doctors perform these methods in a working room, and the individual must be hospitalized.

- *Blood checks*: While program bloodstream tests

only cannot diagnose lung tumour, they could reveal biochemical or metabolic abnormalities in the torso that accompany cancers; for example, *raised levels of calcium mineral or the enzyme alkaline phosphatase may accompany malignancy which is metastatic to the bone fragments.*

Likewise, high degrees of certain enzymes usually present within liver organ cells, including aspartate aminotransferase (AST or SGOT) and alanine aminotransferase (ALT or SGPT), transmission liver organ harm, possibly through the existence of tumour metastatic to the liver organ. One current concentrate of research in the region of lung tumour is the introduction of a bloodstream test to assist in the analysis of lung tumour.

- *Molecular testing*: For advanced NSCLCs, healthcare professionals perform molecular hereditary testing to consider genetic mutations in the tumour. Variations that are accountable for tumour development are drivers' mutations; for instance, *testing may be achieved to find mutations or abnormalities in the epithelial development factor receptor (EGFR) and the anaplastic lymphoma kinase (ALK) genes.* Other genes that may mutate include *MAPK and PIK3.* Specific therapies can be found, which may be given to patients whose tumours have these modifications in their genes.

How Doctors Determine Lung Malignancy Stages?

The stage of the cancer is a way of measuring the extent to which cancer has spread in the torso. Staging consists of an evaluation of cancer's size and its penetration into encircling cells as well as the existence or lack of metastases in the lymph nodes or other organs.

Staging is essential in determining the treating of a particular tumour since lung tumour therapies are aimed toward specific phases. Stage of the cancer is critical in estimating the prognosis of the confirmed patient, with higher-stage malignancies generally using a worse prognosis than lower-stage fatalities.

Doctors could use several testings' to accurately stage lung cancer, which includes; *lab (bloodstream chemistry) exams, X-rays, CT scans, bone scans, MRI scans, and Family pet scans.* Abnormal bloodstream chemistry lab tests may sign the existence of metastases in bone or liver organ, and radiological methods can document how big is a tumour as well as its pass on.

Doctors assign a stage to NSCLC from I to IV to be able of intensity:

- In stage I - the cancer is limited to the lung.

- In stages II and III - the cancer is restricted to the chest *(with bigger and more intrusive tumours categorized as stage III).*

- Stage IV - malignancy has passed on from the upper body to other areas of your body.

Most doctors use a two-tiered system to determine treatment for SCLC:

- Limited-stage (LS) SCLC - identifies cancers that are limited to its part of the source in the upper body.

- <u>In extensive-stage (ES) SCLC</u> - the tumour has passed on beyond the upper body to other areas of your body.

A medical team performs surgery.

What is the Procedure for Lung Cancers?

Treatment for lung malignancy primarily involves *surgery of the tumour, chemotherapy, or rays' therapy, as well as mixtures of the medications*, targeted therapies, and immunotherapy treatments have become more prevalent as well. Your choice about which treatments will be befitting a given specific must look at the location and level of the tumour, as well as the entire health position of the individual.

Much like other malignancies, doctors may prescribe therapy designed to be curative *(removal or eradication of the cancer tumour)* or palliative *(steps that cannot cure cancer but can decrease pain and hurting)*. Doctors may prescribe several kinds of therapy; in such instances, the treatment that is put into enhancing the effects of the principal therapy is known as ***adjuvant therapy***. An excellent example of adjuvant therapy is chemotherapy or radiotherapy implemented after surgery of the tumour so that they can destroy any tumour cells that stays following surgery.

- **Surgery:** Doctors generally perform surgery of the tumour for limited-stage (stage I or sometimes stage II) NSCLC, and it is the treating choice for cancers that haven't pass on beyond the lung. About 10%-35% of lung malignancies can be removed surgically, but removal will not always lead to a cure, because the tumours may currently have passed on and can recur later. Among individuals who have an isolated, slow-growing lung malignancy removed, 25%-40% remain alive five years after medical diagnosis. It's essential to notice that although a tumour may be anatomically ideal for resection, surgery might not be possible if the individual has other serious conditions (such as severe centre or lung disease) that could limit their capability to survive a surgical procedure.

Cosmetic surgeons perform surgery less often with SCLC than with NSCLC because these tumours are less inclined to be localized to 1 area that may be removed.

The medical procedure chosen is dependent upon the scale and located area of the tumour. Doctors must open up the chest wall structure and may execute a wedge resection of the lung (removal of some of 1 lobe), a lobectomy (removal of 1 lobe), or a pneumonectomy (removal of a whole lung). Sometimes lymph nodes around the lungs are also removed (lymphadenectomy). Surgery for lung cancers is a significant surgical procedure that will require general anesthesia, hospitalization, and follow-up look after weeks to weeks. The potential risks of surgery include problems due to blood loss, infection, and issues of general anesthesia.

A male patient gets rays treatment for cancer.

- **Radiation:** Rays therapy goodies both NSCLC and SCLC. Rays therapy uses high-energy X-rays or other styles of rays to eliminate dividing cancer cells. Rays therapy may get as curative therapy, palliative therapy (using lower dosages of rays than with therapeutic therapy), or as adjuvant therapy in mixture with surgery or chemotherapy. Doctors deliver beams either externally, by utilizing a machine that directs rays toward the malignancy, or internally through keeping radioactive chemicals in sealed storage containers within the region of your body where the tumour is localized. Brachytherapy is a term that explains the utilization of a little pellet of radioactive materials placed straight into the tumour or into the airway next to the cancers.

Rays therapy can get if a person refuses surgery, if a tumour has passed on to areas like the lymph nodes or trachea making operation impossible, or if one has other conditions that produce them too sick to endure major surgery. Rays therapy generally only shrinks a tumour or limitations its development when given as a single therapy, yet in 10%-15% of individuals, it leads to long-term remission and palliation of the malignancy. Combining rays' therapy with chemotherapy can further extend success when chemotherapy is given. Someone who has severe lung disease and a lung tumour may not have the ability to get radiotherapy to the lung because the rays can further lower the function of the lungs.

A kind of external ray's therapy called stereotactic radiosurgery, may also be used to take care of solitary brain metastases. In this process, multiple beams of rays via different directions are centred on the tumour over a few moments as the brain is held, set up with a rigid framework. This reduces the dosage of rays that are received by non-cancerous tissues.

For exterior radiation therapy, an activity called simulation is essential preceding to treatment. Using CT scans, computer systems, and specific measurements, simulation maps out the precise location where the rays will be shipped, called the procedure field or slot. The external ray's treatment itself generally is performed 4 or 5 days weekly for many weeks.

SCLC often spreads to the brain, sometimes people who have SCLC that is responding well to treatment are treated with rays' therapy to the top to take care of the very early spread to the brain (called *micrometastasis*) that's not yet detectable with CT or MRI scans and hasn't however produced symptoms. That is known as prophylactic brain rays. Brain rays' therapy can cause short-term memory space problems, exhaustion, nausea, and other aspect effects.

Radiation therapy will not carry the dangers of significant surgery, but it can have unpleasant part effects, including exhaustion and insufficient energy. A lower life expectancy white bloodstream cell count number (making a person more vulnerable to contamination) and low bloodstream platelet levels (making bloodstream clotting more challenging and leading to excessive blood loss) can also occur with rays' therapy. If the digestive organs are in the field subjected to rays, patients may experience nausea, throwing up, or diarrhea. Rays therapy can irritate your skin; the region that is treated, but this discomfort generally improves as time passes after treatment is finished.

A vial of chemotherapy drugs with fine needles.

- **Chemotherapy:** Both NSCLC and SCLC may be treated with chemotherapy. Chemotherapy identifies the administration of drugs that stop the development of malignancy cells by eliminating them or avoiding them from dividing. Chemotherapy may get only, as an adjuvant to medical therapy, or in mixture with radiotherapy. While lots of chemotherapeutic drugs have been developed, the course of medicines known as platinum-based drugs has been the very best in the treatment of lung malignancies.

Chemotherapy is the treatment choice for some SCLC since these tumours are usually widespread in the torso when they may be diagnosed. Only fifty percent of people who've SCLC survive for a few months without chemotherapy. With chemotherapy, their success time is increased up to four- to fivefold. Chemotherapy only is not especially useful in dealing with NSCLC; however, when NSCLC has metastasized, it can prolong success often.

Chemotherapy may gotten as pills, as an intravenous infusion, or as a mixture of both. Chemotherapy treatments tend to be given within an outpatient establishing. A combination of drugs is given in some treatments, called cycles, over weeks to weeks, with breaks among cycles. Regrettably, the drugs found in chemotherapy also usually destroy dividing cells in the torso, leading to unpleasant aspect results.

Damage to bloodstream cells can lead to increased susceptibility to attacks and problems with bloodstream clotting (blood loss or bruising easily). Other part results include exhaustion, weight loss, hair thinning, nausea, throwing up, diarrhea, and mouth area sores. The medial side effects of chemotherapy differ based on the dose and mixture of drugs used and could also change from person to person. Medications have been developed that can treat or prevent lots of the aspect effects of chemotherapy. The medial side results generally disappear through the recovery stage of the procedure or following its completion.

- **<u>Targeted therapy</u>:** Molecularly targeted therapy

involves the administration of drugs that have been recognized to work in subsets of patients whose tumours have specific genetic changes (driver mutations) that promote tumour growth.

- **EGFR-targeted therapies:** The drugs erlotinib *(Tarceva), afatinib (Gilotrif), and gefitinib (Iressa)* are types of so-called targeted drugs that more specifically target cancer cells, leading to less harm to healthy cells than general chemotherapeutic agents. Erlotinib, gefitinib, and afatinib focus on a protein called *the epidermal development factor receptor (EGFR)* that is important to advertise the department of cells. The gene encoding this protein is often mutated of non-small-cell lung tumour, developing a mutation that stimulates tumour development. Mutations in the EGFR gene are more prevalent in malignancies in women and individuals who have never smoked.

Drugs that focus on the EGFR receptor sometimes go wrong after a period, which is recognized as a level of resistance to the medication. The level of resistance often occurs because the cancers have developed a new mutation in the same gene, and a typical exemplary case of this is the so-called EGFR T790M mutation. Some newer EGFR-targeted drugs also work against cells with the T790M mutation, including *osimertinib (Tagrisso)*. *Necitumumab (Portrazza)* is another medication that focuses on EGFR. It could be used along with chemotherapy as the first treatment in people who have advanced NSCLC of the squamous cell type.

- **<u>Other targeted therapies</u>:** Other targeted drugs can be found that focus on other drivers' mutations. Types of these other targeted therapies are the ALK tyrosine kinase inhibitor drugs; *crizotinib (Xalkori), alectinib (Alecensa), brigatinib (Alunbrig), and ceritinib (Zykadia)* that are found in patients whose tumours come with an abnormality of the ALK gene as the driver's mutation. A few of these drugs can also be helpful for individuals whose cancers come with a defect of the gene known as ROS1.

The gene known as **_BRAF_** may also be abnormal in lung

cancers leading to the production of BRAF protein that promotes cancer's growth. Dabrafenib (Tafinlar) is a kind of medication known as a BRAF inhibitor and episodes the BRAF proteins straight. Trametinib (Mekinist) is a MEK inhibitor since its chapters MEK protein that is related to BRAF protein. These can be utilized for patients with tumours which have irregular BRAF genes.

Other efforts at targeted therapy include drugs known as *antiangiogenesis drugs*, which stop the introduction of new arteries within a malignancy; without adequate bloodstream to provide oxygen-carrying blood, the malignancy cells will pass away. The antiangiogenic medication bevacizumab (Avastin) also has been found to prolong success in advanced lung tumour when it's added to the typical chemotherapy routine. Bevacizumab is given intravenously every 2-3 weeks. However, since this medication may cause blood loss, it isn't befitting use in lung cancer patients who are paying bloodstream, if the lung malignancy has passed on to the brain, or in folks who are getting anticoagulation therapy ("bloodstream leaner" medications). Bevacizumab is not found in situations of squamous cell tumour since it leads to blood loss from this kind of lung cancer. Ramucirumab (Cyramza) is another angiogenesis inhibitor you can use to take care of advanced non-small-cell lung malignancy.

- **Immunotherapy:** Immunotherapy may be a highly effective option for a few patients with advanced lung malignancies. Immunotherapy drugs work by conditioning the experience of the disease fighting capability against tumour cells. The immunotherapy drugs nivolumab (Opdivo) and pembrolizumab (Keytruda) are checkpoint inhibitors that focus on checkpoints or areas that control the immune system response and promote the immune system response. Both of these drugs focus on the PD-1 proteins, which strengthens the immune system response against malignancies. Atezolizumab (Tecentriq) and durvalumab (Imfinzi) are types of medicines that focus on PD-L1, a protein related to PD-1 that is available on some tumour cells and immune system cells.

- **Radiofrequency ablation (RFA):** Radiofrequency

ablation may also be used for small tumours located close to the lungs instead of surgery, particularly instances of early-stage lung tumour. In this kind of treatment, a needle is put through your skin to the cancers, usually under assistance by CT scanning. Radiofrequency (electric) energy is then sent to the end of the needle, where it produces warmth in the tissue, eliminating the cancerous tissues and shutting small arteries supplying the malignancy. Studies show that treatment can prolong success, much like surgery, when used to take care of first stages of lung tumour but with no dangers of major surgery and the long-term recovery time associated with primary surgical treatments.

- **<u>Experimental therapies</u>:** Since no therapy happens to be available that is entirely effective in treating lung cancer, patients may be offered lots of new therapies that remain the experimental stage, and therefore doctors do not yet have sufficient information to choose whether these therapies should become accepted types of treatment for lung cancer. New drugs or new combos of drugs are examined in so-called medical trials, which are studies that measure the performance of new medications in comparison to those treatments already in everyday use.

Newer types of immunotherapy are being analyzed that involve the utilization of vaccine-related therapies that try to make use of the body's disease-fighting capability to directly battle malignancy cells. Lung cancer treatment vaccines are being researched in clinical tests.

What's the Prognosis and Life Span of Lung Malignancy?

The prognosis of lung cancer identifies the opportunity for cure or prolongation of life (survival) and depends upon where the cancer is situated, how big is cancer, the existence of symptoms, the kind of lung cancer, and the entire health status of the individual.

SCLC gets the most aggressive development of most

lung malignancies, with a median success time of only two to four a few months after analysis when untreated. (That's, by two to four weeks, half of most patients have passed away). However, SCLC is also the kind of lung tumour most attentive to rays' therapy and chemotherapy. Because SCLC spreads quickly, and its usually disseminated during medical diagnosis, methods such as surgery or localized rays' therapy are less effective in dealing with this kind of lung cancer. When chemotherapy is utilized by itself or in mixture with other methods, success time can be extended four- to fivefold; however, of most patients with SCLC, only 5%-10% remain alive five years after analysis. The majority of those who survive have limited-stage SCLC before treatment.

In non-small-cell lung malignancy (NSCLC), the most crucial prognostic factor is the stage (extent of spread) of the tumour during medical diagnosis. Results of standard treatment are usually weak in every; however, the smallest of malignancies that may be surgically removed. In stage I fatalities that may be removed entirely surgically, five-year success approaches 75%. Rays therapy can create a remedy in a little minority of patients with NSCLC and leads to alleviation of symptoms generally in most patients. In advanced-stage disease, chemotherapy offers moderate improvements in success, although rates of overall success are reduced.

The entire prognosis for lung cancer is weak in comparison to various other cancers. Success rates for lung malignancy are generally less than those for some cancers, with a standard five-year success rate for lung tumour around 17% in comparison to 65% for cancer of the colon, 91% for breasts tumour, 81% for bladder cancers, and over 99% for prostate malignancy.

Can You Prevent Lung Tumour?

Cessation of smoking and eliminating contact with tobacco smoke cigarettes is the most crucial measure that can prevent lung cancers. Many products, such as nicotine gum, nicotine sprays, or nicotine inhalers, may be beneficial to people attempting to give up smoking. Minimizing contact with passive smoking is a useful precautionary measure. Utilizing a home radon test package can identify and invite modification of increased radon levels in the house. Methods that allow early recognition of cancers, like the low-dose CT scan, also may be of value in the identification of small malignancies that may be cured by operative resection and avoided from becoming wide-spread, incurable metastatic malignancy.

Chapter 2

Causes of lung cancer

Smoking causes nearly all lung malignancies, both in smokers and in people subjected to secondhand smoke cigarettes. However, lung tumour also occurs in people who never smoked and in those who never really had prolonged contact with secondhand smoke cigarettes. In such cases, there could be no apparent reason for lung cancers.

How Smoking Causes Lung Cancer

Doctors believe smoking causes lung malignancy by damaging the cells collection in the lungs. When you inhale tobacco smoke, which is filled with cancer-causing chemicals (carcinogens), changes in the lung tissues start almost immediately.

At first, the body might be able to repair this harm, but with the repetition of these, healthy cells that range your lungs are progressively damaged. As time passes, the injury causes cells to do something abnormally, and finally, malignancy may develop.

Types of Lung Cancer

Doctors separate lung tumour into two significant types, predicated on the looks of lung cancer cells under the microscope. Your physician makes treatment decisions predicated on which significant kind of lung malignancy you have.

Both general types of lung cancer include:

- ***Small cell lung cancer***: Small cell lung tumour occurs almost specifically in heavy smokers, and it is less common than non-small cell lung cancers.

- ***Non-small cell lung malignancy***: Non-small cell lung tumour can be an umbrella term for several types of lung malignancies that behave similarly. Non-small cell lung malignancies include squamous cell carcinoma, adenocarcinoma, and large cell carcinoma.

Risk factors

Several factors may boost your threat of lung cancer; some risk factors can be managed, for example, by giving up smoking.

Risk factors for lung cancers include:

- **Smoking**: Your threat of lung malignancy increases with the number of smokes you smoke every day, and the number of years you have burned. Giving up at any age group can significantly decrease your threat of developing lung tumour.

- **Contact with secondhand smoke cigarettes**: Even though you don't smoke cigarettes, your threat of lung cancers increases if you are subjected to secondhand smoke cigarettes.

- **Contact with radon gas**: Radon is made by the natural break down of uranium in-ground, rock, and drinking water that eventually becomes an area of the air you inhale. Unsafe degrees of radon can accumulate in virtually any building, including homes.

- **Contact with asbestos and other carcinogens**: Place of work contact with asbestos and other chemicals recognized to cause malignancy, such as arsenic, chromium, and nickel, can also increase your threat of developing lung tumour, particularly if you're a cigarette smoker.

- **Genealogy of lung cancers**: People who have a mother or father, sibling, or child with lung malignancy have an elevated risk of the condition.

- **Complications**: Lung tumour can cause complications, such as:

    - *Shortness of breathing*: People who have lung cancers can experience shortness of breath if cancer develops to stop the significant airways. Lung malignancy can also cause the liquid to accumulate around the lungs, which makes it harder for the affected lung to increase ultimately when you inhale.

- *Coughing up blood vessels*: Lung tumour can cause blood loss in the airways, which can make you cough up bloodstream (hemoptysis). Sometimes blood loss may become severe. Treatments can be found to control blood loss.

- *Pain*: Advanced lung cancers that spread to the liner of the lung or even to another section of the body, like a bone, can distress. Tell your physician if you have pain, as many treatments can be found to regulate pain.

- *The liquid in the upper body (pleural effusion)*: Lung malignancy can cause the liquid to build up in the area that surrounds the affected lung in the upper body cavity (pleural space).

- *Liquid accumulating in the upper body can cause shortness of breathing*: Treatments can be found to drain the fluid from your upper body and decrease the risk that pleural effusion will happen again.

- **<u>Tumor that spreads to other areas of your body (metastasis)</u>**: Lung tumour often spreads (metastasizes) to other areas of your body, like the brain and the bone fragments.

Cancers that spreads can cause distress, nausea, headaches, or other signs or symptoms depending on what body organ is affected. Once lung cancers pass on beyond the lungs, it's generally not curable. Treatments can be found to decrease signs or symptoms and also to help your home is longer.

Prevention of Lung Cancer

There is no sure way to avoid lung cancer; nevertheless, you can lessen your risk if you:

- ***Don't smoke***: If you have never smoked, don't start. Speak to your children about not smoking to learn how to avoid this significant risk factor for lung malignancy. Begin discussions about the risks of smoking with your kids early so that they learn how to respond to peer pressure.

Quitting smoke reduces your threat of lung tumour, even

if you have smoked for a long time. Speak to your doctor about strategies to stop-smoking. Options include alternative nicotine products, medications, and organizations.

- *Avoid secondhand smoke cigarettes*: If you live or utilize a cigarette smoker, urge her or him to quit or instead ask her or him to smoke cigarettes outside. Avoid areas where people smoke cigarettes, such as pubs and restaurants, and look for smoke-free options.

- *Test your home for radon thoroughly*: Have the radon levels in your house checked, mainly if you reside in a location where radon may be considered a problem. High radon levels can be remedied to help your home be safer. For information on radon screening, contact your neighbourhood department of general public health or an area section of the American Lung Association.

- *Avoid carcinogens at the job*: Take precautions to safeguard yourself from contact with toxic chemicals at the position. Follow your employer's safety measures. *For instance, if you are given a nose and mouth mask for safety, always use it.* Ask your physician what more you can do to safeguard yourself at the job. Your threat of lung harm from the place of work carcinogens raises if you smoke cigarettes.

- *Eat a diet plan full of fruits & vegetables*: Select a nutritious diet with several vegetables & fruits; food resources of nutrients and vitamins are best. Avoid taking large dosages of vitamin supplements in tablet form, as they might be harmful. For example, researchers hoping to lessen the chance of lung cancers in heavy smokers gave them beta carotene supplements. Results demonstrated the supplements increased the likelihood of malignancy in smokers.

- *Exercise most times of the week*: Unless you exercise regularly, begin slowly. Make an effort to use most times of the week.

Chapter 3

Symptoms of Lung Cancer

In people who have lung cancer, symptoms only occur when the condition has already reached a later stage. However, many people may notice symptoms that they may think are related to a less severe and acute illness.

Types of these medical indications include:

- Appetite loss.

- Changes in someone's tone of voice, such as hoarseness.

- Regular chest infections, such as bronchitis or pneumonia.

- Lingering coughing that may begin to get worse.

- Shortness of breath.

- Unexplained headaches.

- Weight loss.

- Wheezing.

A person could also experience more severe symptoms associated with lung cancer; included in these are the rigid upper body or bone pain or paying blood.

Diagnosis

If a health care provider identifies a suspicious lesion on lung cancer testing, or one is experiencing symptoms that could indicate lung cancer, several diagnostic tests can be found to confirm.

Examples included in these are:

- **Imaging Studies:** Computed tomography (CT) and positron emission tomography (Family pet) scans might uncover regions of lung cells with cancers. Bone scans can also show cancerous growths. Doctors could also use these scans to monitor the improvement of treatment or even to ensure cancer hasn't returned, carrying out a procedure. MRI scan (Imaging can help screen a lung tumour or monitor the improvement of treatment).

- **Cells Sampling:** If a health care provider identifies a suspicious lesion with imaging research, they could recommend going for a test of lung tissues to check for potentially cancerous cells; there are different ways to have this test, and the technique often depends upon the positioning of the lesion. One of these is whenever a doctor performs a *bronchoscopy* that involves inserting a particularly thin, lighted range with a camera on the flesh; this can help the physician to start seeing the lesion and then to acquire samples.

Less accessible lesions in the lungs may necessitate a far more invasive medical procedure to eliminate lung cells, such as thoracoscopy or video-assisted thoracic surgery.

- **Lab Screening:** A health care provider could also order sputum tests or blood assessment to check on for the existence of lung malignancy; a doctor uses these details to know what kind of lung tumour may be there, and exactly how advanced the condition has become.

The need for early diagnosis

Early diagnosis of lung cancer can be lifesaving; this is because lung cancers cells can be developed in some regions of the body even before health care provider detects them in the lungs; which makes dealing with the disease a lot more complicated. Sometimes, a health care provider will recommend lung malignancy screenings to the patient; they are performed utilizing a low-dose CT scanning device.

Based on the *American Lung Association*, people who may be applicants for lung cancers screenings are those who:

- Are between 55 and 80 years having a 30 pack-year background of smoking, meaning they smoked one pack each day for 30 years or two packages for 15 years.

- Are present smokers or smoker that has quit within days gone by 15 years.

Insurance will most likely cover this testing if a person

matches all these requirements; however, people should talk with their insurance provider before registering for lung cancer testing.

How does a health care provider diagnose cancer?

Staging of Cancer

The stage of cancer indicates what lengths they have spread through your body and its severity. This classification helps clinicians support and immediate treatment to discover the best results. Each stage determines if malignancy has or hasn't passed on (to close by lymph nodes), it could also look at the quantity and size of the tumours.

The *lymph nodes* are an area of the lymphatic system, which connects to all of that other body; if the tumour gets to these nodes, it can metastasize, or pass on further, becoming more threatening.

Staging for lung malignancy is incredibly complex and considerable, with several sub-groups within each stage. In the beginning, clinicians divide it into small cell and non-small cell classifications.

Staging definitions can vary greatly, but doctors typically stage non-small cell lung cancers using the tumour size and the spread to steer them in the following way:

- **Occult/concealed:** Cancer will not show on imaging scans, but cancerous cells might come in the phlegm or mucus and could have reached other areas of your body.

- **Stage 0:** The physician sees abnormal cells only in the very best levels of cells coating the airways.

- **Stage I:** A tumour is rolling out in the lung, but is under 5 centimetres (cm) and hasn't spread to other areas of your body.

- **Stage II:** The tumour is smaller than 5cm and may have passed on to the lymph nodes in the region of the lung, or lower than 7cm and pass on to nearby cells, however, not lymph nodes.

- **Stage III:** Tumor has passed on to the lymph nodes and reached other areas of the lung and surrounding area.

- **Stage IV:** Cancers has passed on to distant areas of the body, like the bone fragments or brain.

Small cell lung cancer has its categories, limited and intensive, discussing whether the disease has passed on within or beyond your lungs.

Treatment

Treatments for lung malignancy depend on it is location and stage, as well as the entire health of the person. Surgery and rays are the most typical methods of treating lung tumour, but other treatments can be found. For instance, doctors often treat small cell lung cancers with chemotherapy.

Possible treatments include:

- **Surgery:** A health care provider may operate to eliminate cancerous lung tissues and cells in the encompassing areas where malignancy may have a pass on. This sometimes entails removing a lobe or large section of the lung in operation called a lobectomy.

In severe cases, the surgeon may remove a lung in its entirety. An individual can live without a lung, but being in good health before surgery helps to improve results after lung removal.

- **_Chemotherapy_**: This treatment uses drugs to shrink or eradicate tumour cells; these medications focus on quickly dividing cells, making them perfect for treating cancer.

Chemotherapy treatment has a far more significant effect on cancers, which have passed on to various areas of your body and need a body-wide attack. However, chemotherapy is a robust intervention and can have side results, including extreme nausea and weight reduction.

- **_Radiation therapy_**: This process uses high-energy rays to get rid of cancerous cells. A health care provider could also use rays to reduce a tumour before getting rid of it surgically.

Radiation therapy is principally useful in fatalities that occur in a single location and also have not spread.

- ***Targeted therapy*:** This is the use of particular medications that specifically target a specific behaviour in cancer cells. For example, drugs that stop cancer cells from multiplying.

Lung malignancy treatment often involves the collaboration of doctors in many areas. These specialists can include:

- Surgeons.

- Radiation oncologists.

- Specialists in lung treatment called pulmonologists.

- Pulmonary therapists.

Chapter 4

Phases of Lung Cancer

Cancer stages show what lengths the tumour has passed on and helped guide treatment. The opportunity of successful or curative treatment is a lot higher when lung cancer is diagnosed and treated in the first stages before it spreads because lung cancers don't cause apparent symptoms in the last stages, analysis often employs it has passed on.

Non-small cell lung malignancy has four primary levels:

Stage 1: Malignancy is situated in the lung, but it hasn't spread beyond your lung.

Stage 2: Tumor is situated in the lung and closes by lymph nodes.

Stage 3: Malignancy is within the lung and lymph nodes in the centre of the chest.

Stage 3A: Cancers are situated in lymph nodes, but only on a single part of the upper body where the tumour first started growing.

Stage 3B: Malignancy has passed on to lymph nodes on the contrary aspect of the upper body or even to lymph nodes above the collarbone.

Stage 4: Tumor has passed on to both lungs, into the area across the lungs, or even to distant organs.

Small-cell lung cancers (SCLC) has two main phases; in the limited stage, malignancy is situated in only one lung or close by lymph nodes on a single part of the upper body.

The comprehensive stage means cancer has spread:

- Throughout one lung.
- To the contrary lung.
- To lymph nodes on the contrary side.
- To fluid throughout the lung.
- To bone marrow.
- To distant organs

During diagnosis, 2 out of 3 people who have SCLC are already in a critical stage.

Lung malignancy and back again pain

Back pain is rather joint in the overall population. It's possible to have lung tumour and unrelated back yet pain. A lot of people with back pain don't have lung cancers; not everyone with lung malignancy gets back pain, but many do. For a lot of, back pain is the main symptom of lung tumour.

Back pain can be because of the pressure of large tumours growing in the lungs. Additionally, it may mean that cancers have passed on to your backbone or ribs. Since it expands, a cancerous tumour can cause compression of the spinal cord.

That can lead to neurologic deterioration leading to:

- Weakness of the legs and arms.

- Numbness or lack of feeling in the hip and legs and feet.

- Urinary and bowel incontinence.

- Disturbance with the spine blood supply.

With no treatment, back pain caused by cancer will continue steadily to worsen. Back pain may improve if treatment such as surgery, rays, or chemotherapy can effectively remove or reduce the tumour. Also, your physician may use corticosteroids or prescription pain relievers, such as acetaminophen and non-steroidal anti-inflammatory drugs (NSAIDs). For more serious pain, opioids such as morphine or oxycodone may be needed.

Risk Factors for Lung Cancer

The most significant risk factor for lung cancer is smoking; which includes *smoking, cigars, and pipes*. Cigarette products contain a large number of toxic substances.

Based on the Centers for Disease Control and Prevention (CDC) Respected Source, cigarette smokers are 15 to 30 times much more likely to get lung malignancy than non-smokers. The much longer you smoke, the higher the opportunity of developing lung tumour. Giving up smoking can lower that risk.

Sucking in secondhand smoke cigarettes is also a significant risk factor. Each year in America, about 7,300 people who've never smoked pass away from lung cancers triggered by secondhand smoke cigarettes.

Contact with radon, a naturally occurring gas, boosts your threat of lung malignancy. Radon increases from the bottom, entering structures through small splits. It's the best reason behind lung tumour in non-smokers. A straightforward home test can let you know if the amount of radon in your house is hazardous.

Your threat of developing lung malignancy is higher if you're subjected to toxins such as asbestos or diesel exhaust at work.

Other risk factors include:

- Genealogy of lung cancer.

- Personal history of lung cancer, particularly if you're a smoker.

- Earlier radiation therapy to the chest.

Lung Cancers and Smoking

Not absolutely all smokers get lung malignancy, rather than everyone that has lung tumour is a cigarette smoker. But there's without a doubt that smoking is the most significant risk factor, leading to 9 out of 10 trusted source lung cancers. Furthermore, tobacco, cigar, and tube smoking are also associated with lung cancer. The greater and longer you smoke, the more significant your potential for developing lung cancer.

You don't need to be a smoker to be affected; Sucking in other people's smoke cigarettes increases the threat of lung tumour. Based on the *Centers for Disease Control and Avoidance (CDC)* - Trusted Source, secondhand smoke cigarettes are accountable for about 7,300 lung cancer deaths every year in America. Tobacco products contain much more than 7,000 chemicals, with least 70 are recognized to cause cancer.

When you inhale cigarette smoke, this combination of chemicals is delivered right to your lungs, where it immediately starts leading to damage. The lungs can usually repair harm at first; however, the continued influence on lung tissue becomes harder to control. That's when broken cells can mutate and develop uncontrollably.

The chemicals you inhale also enter your bloodstream and are carried through your body, increasing the chance of other styles of cancer. Former smokers remain vulnerable to developing lung malignancy, but quitting can lower that risk considerably within a decade of stopping, the chance of dying from lung cancer drops by half.

Facts and figures about Lung Cancer

Lung cancers are the most typical malignancy in the world. Based on the American Lung Association, there have been 2.1 million new cases in 2018, as well as 1.8 million fatalities from lung cancer. The most frequent type is non-small cell lung cancer (NSCLC), accounting for 80 to 85 percent of most cases, based on the Lung Cancer Alliance.

Small-cell lung tumour (SCLC) represents about 15 to 20 percent of lung malignancies. During analysis, 2 out of 3 individuals with SCLC are actually in the comprehensive stage. Anyone can get lung cancers, but smoking or contact with secondhand smoke cigarettes is associated with about 90 percent of lung malignancy cases. Based on the Centers for Disease Control and Prevention (CDC) Trusted Source, cigarette smokers are 15 to 30 times much more likely to get lung cancer than non-smokers.

In America, every year, about 7,300 people who never smoked die from lung cancer caused by secondhand smoke. Former smokers remain vulnerable to developing lung tumour, but quitting can significantly lower that risk. Within a decade of stopping, the chance of dying from lung cancers drops by half-Trusted Source.

Tobacco products contain much more than 7,000 chemicals. At least 70 are known carcinogens. Based on *the US Environmental Protection Agency (EPA),* radon is accountable for about 21,000 lung malignancy deaths each year in the USA. About 2,900 of those deaths take place among individuals who have never smoked; black people are in higher threat of developing and about to die from lung tumour than other racial and cultural groups.

Chapter 5

What are pulmonary nodules?

A pulmonary nodule is a little around or oval-shaped development in the lung. It could also be called an "I'm all over this the lung" or a "gold coin lesion." Pulmonary nodules are smaller than 3 centimetres (around 1.2 INS) in diameter. If the development is more significant than that, it is named a pulmonary mass, and it is much more likely to represent a malignancy when compared to a nodule.

How common are pulmonary nodules?

Many pulmonary nodules are uncovered every year during chest X-rays or CT scans. Most nodules are non-cancerous (harmless). A solitary pulmonary nodule is available on up to 0.2% of most upper body X-rays films. Lung nodules are available on up to fifty percent of most lung CT scans. Risk factors for malignant pulmonary nodules add a background of smoking and old age.

What can cause pulmonary nodules?

You will find two main types of pulmonary nodules: *malignant (cancerous) and benign (non-cancerous)*. Over 90% of pulmonary nodules that are smaller than two centimetres (around 3/4) in diameter are mild.

Benign pulmonary nodules can have a multitude of causes. Most are the consequence of swelling in the lung, consequently of contamination or disease-producing irritation in the torso. The nodule may represent a dynamic process or be the consequence of scar tissue formation related to prior swelling. Benign developmental lesions could also show up as nodules.

Attacks - most attacks that appear much like pulmonary nodules are relatively lazy and frequently not active. For example, *mycobacterium, such as mycobacterium tuberculosis or mycobacterium avium intracellulare, and fungal attacks such as aspergillosis, histoplasmosis, coccidiomycosis, and cryptococcosis*. Swelling related to attacks often form what is termed a granuloma; granuloma is a little clump of cells that form when lung tissues become swollen. Granulomas form when the disease fighting capability isolates substances it considers international. More often than not, granulomas happen in the lungs; however; they could also develop in other areas of your body, they can become calcified as time passes, as calcium will gather in the recovery tissue.

Non-infectious factors behind harmless inflammatory lung nodules – Non-infectious disorders such as *sarcoidosis, granulomatosis with polyangiitis (GPA), and arthritis rheumatoid* also show themselves with granulomas forming in the lungs.

Neoplasms - Neoplasms are abnormal growths that may be benign or malignant. Types of harmless tumours include:

- Fibroma (a lump of fibrous connective cells).

- Hamartoma (an abnormal grouping of healthy cells).

- Neurofibroma (a lump composed of nerve tissues).

- Blastoma (a rise composed of immature cells)

Types of malignant tumours include:

- Lung cancer.

- Lymphoma (a rise is containing lymphoid cells).

- Carcinoid (a small, slow-growing cancerous tumour).

- Sarcoma (a tumour comprising connective tissues).

- Metastatic tumours (tumours which have distributed to the lungs from cancer in another area of the body).

What are the symptoms of pulmonary nodules?

Usually, there are no symptoms associated with pulmonary nodules. If presented, signs would be related to the problem that resulted in the nodule developing. If the nodule is from lung cancer, the individual is often without symptoms but may have a new cough, or coughing up blood.

More often than not, an individual is unaware that he/she

has a lung nodule until an upper body X-ray or computed tomography check out (CT check) of the lungs is conducted.

How is Pulmonary nodules Diagnosed?

Though most lung nodules aren't malignant, it is vital that those representing cancer are recognized early in their course, when they may be curable.

- <u>Upper body X-rays and CT scans</u>: Usually, the first indication a pulmonary nodule exists is an area on the lung that presents through to an upper-body X-ray or a CT check out. These assessments are usually done whenever a person views the physician for a respiratory system illness.

If the X-ray film or CT check indicates there's a pulmonary nodule, your physician will ask you about your health background, including whether you experienced cancer before. She or he would want to know whether you are a cigarette smoker or a former cigarette smoker and about any contact with environmental chemicals that may be toxic.

The doctor can look at the X-ray to judge the scale and form of the nodule, its location, and its general appearance. Solitary pulmonary nodules seen on upper body x-rays are usually at least 8 to 10 millimetres in diameter. If they're smaller than that, these are improbable to be noticeable on an upper-body X-ray; the more significant the nodule is, and the higher irregularly formed it is, the much more likely it is usually to be cancerous. Those positioned in the upper servings of the lung are also much more likely to be cancerous.

When you have any older upper body X-rays, you should let your physician take a look at them to look for the development rate of the nodule. Generally, Nodules with a slower or faster development rate are less inclined to be cancerous. Your physician may advise that you undergo a CT check out to secure a more descriptive image of the nodule, or your nodule may have first been determined with a CT check. CT scans can provide information about the precise top features of the nodule, including its form, size, location, and inner density. CT scans are more accurate than upper body x-rays in identifying the type of the nodule. A CT scan will get tiny nodules, no more than 1-2 mm in diameter.

If the nodule is small enough or if its features suggest an extremely low likelihood it signifies cancer, your physician will probably follow the nodule as time passes with repeated chest imaging. If the nodule will not grow as time passes, it is verified to be harmless. If a regarding pace of development is mentioned, then additional evaluation would be recommended. The period between scans and the space of follow-up depends upon how big is the nodule and the chance of malignancy.

- <u>Positron emission tomography (Family pet)</u>: A Family pet checks out can also help to discover if a nodule is malignant or benign. A Family pet scan runs on the radiolabeled material such as blood sugar that is assimilated by the nodule, and an image of the nodule's metabolic activity level. Malignant cells have faster metabolic rates than healthy cells, so they might need more energy and therefore absorb more of the radiolabeled compound.

Nodules can light on Family pet imagine if they're malignant or when there is energetic inflammation. We must be cautious with your pet scan interpretation when someone has nodules smaller than 8-10 mm because they're not seen well by Family pet imaging.

- Biopsy: A biopsy is an operation in which a little tissue test is taken off the nodule so that it can be examined under a microscope. It might be performed when other checks are inconclusive to eliminate the chance of development in malignant.

You can find two ways, in short supply of going right through surgery, to gather samples from lung tissue. The technique used depends upon the scale and located area of the nodule, as well as the comfort of the medical team with these methods.

- Bronchoscopy: This process is utilized if it seems the nodule can be reached through the deep breathing tubes. It runs on the bronchoscope, which is a slim, lighted, flexible pipe that may be inserted into the mouth area or nasal area and through the windpipe (trachea) into the bronchus (airway) of the lung. The bronchoscope has a tiny camera at its end. Biopsy tools can be exceeded through the camera to attain the nodule.

- <u>Needle biopsy (also called transthoracic needle aspiration)</u>: This test is most successful when the nodule is towards the advantage of the lung, close to the upper body wall structure. A needle is put through the upper body wall and into the nodule, usually under the assistance of the CT scan.

If the nodule has an extremely concerning appearance or growth design, or it somewhat concerns and its nature struggles to be clarified by the tests mentioned above, the best step may be to eliminate the nodule. This will explain its character while dealing with it. This involves the individual be fit enough to endure the surgery.

How are Pulmonary nodules Treated?

If the pulmonary nodule is benign, it usually will not require treatment. If active infection is available or illness of inflammation in the torso is diagnosed, the procedure would be predicated on the condition discovered and the symptoms that can be found.

If the nodule is malignant, there will not look like any spread of cancer, and the individual is fit, then your cancer should be surgically removed. If a nonsurgical biopsy of the nodule with high concern for malignancy is performed and the email address details are inconclusive, it is strongly recommended that the nodule be studied out.

Surgical ways to remove pulmonary nodules include:

- Thoracotomy: This process is considered open up lung surgery. A slice is manufactured in the wall structure of the upper body to get rid of bits of diseased lung cells. Patients will often have to stay in a healthcare facility for a couple of days after the procedure. The mortality risk is low. When possible, a mini-thoracotomy that is less intrusive may be performed.

- Video-Assisted Thoracoscopy: This process runs on the thorascope, a versatile tube with a smaller camera on its end. The thorascope is placed through a little cut into the upper body wall structure. The camera allows the physician to see a graphic of the nodule on the television screen. This system takes a smaller slice and a shorter recovery time, when compared to a thoracotomy.

How can malignant pulmonary nodules be prevented?

*The ultimate way to avoid having a malignant pulmonary nodule is to **give up smoking if you are a smoker**.*

Chapter 6

Lung Nodules and Benign Lung Tumour

If you have received the news that your lung contains something "suspicious," this can be a way to obtain great distress. The very first thing that will come to mind is a feared word - **cancer**. Often, though, a lung nodule is benign, which means that it isn't cancer. A difficult part is waiting around rather than knowing; here's information that could make you wait around just a tiny bit easier.

What Exactly Are Benign Lung Nodules and Benign Lung Tumours?

A nodule is an "I'm all over this the lung," seen with an X-ray or computed tomography (CT) check out. A nodule turns up on about one Atlanta divorce attorney, 500 upper body X-rays. Healthy lung cells surround this small circular or solid oval overgrowth of tissues. It might be an individual or solitary pulmonary nodule. Or, you might have multiple nodules.

Your lung nodule is much more likely to be benign if:

- You are younger than age 40.

- You are a non-smoker.

- There is undoubtedly calcium in the nodule.

- The nodule is small.

A benign lung tumour can be an abnormal development of cells that acts no purpose and is available never to be cancerous. Harmless lung tumours may grow from many different constructions in the lung. Identifying whether a nodule is a benign tumour or an early on stage of malignancy is vital. That's because early recognition and treatment of lung tumour can significantly improve your survival.

What are the Symptoms of Benign Lung Nodules and Tumours?

Benign lung nodules and tumours usually cause no symptoms; that is why they are nearly always found accidentally on the upper body X-ray or CT scan. However, they could lead to symptoms like these:

- Wheezing.

- Coughing that is maintained or paying blood.

- Shortness of breath.

- Fever, particularly if pneumonia exists

What Are the Sources of Benign Lung Nodules and Tumours?

The sources of harmless lung tumours and nodules are poorly understood. However, in general, they often derive from problems like;

Inflammation from attacks such as:

- An infectious fungus (histoplasmosis, coccidioidomycosis, cryptococcosis, or aspergillosis, for example).

- Tuberculosis (TB).

- A lung abscesses.

- Circular pneumonia (uncommon in adults)

Inflammation from non-infectious causes such as:

- Rheumatoid arthritis.

- Wegener granulomatosis.

- Sarcoidosis.

Congenital disabilities like a lung cyst or other lung malformation; these are a few of the more prevalent types of benign lung tumours:

- Hamartomas are the most typical kind of benign lung tumour and the 3rd most common reason behind solitary pulmonary nodules; these company marble-like tumours are made of tissues from the lung's coating as well as cells such as excess fat and cartilage. They're usually situated in the periphery of the lung.

- Bronchial adenomas constitute about half of most harmless lung tumours. They may be a diverse band of tumours that arise from mucous glands and ducts of the windpipe or large airways of the lung. A mucous gland adenoma can be an example of a genuine harmless bronchial adenoma.

Rare neoplasms can include chondromas, fibromas, or lipomas -- harmless tumours composed of connective tissues or fat.

How are Benign Lung Nodules and Tumours Diagnosed?

How does your physician know if a lung nodule is benign? Furthermore, to going for background and performing a physical exam, your physician may "watch" a nodule, taking repeated X-rays throughout 2 yrs. Or much longer if the nodule is smaller than 6 millimetres as well as your risk is low. If the nodule remains the same size for at least 2 yrs., it is known as harmless. That's because harmless lung nodules grow gradually, if. Alternatively, cancerous nodules, usually, double in proportions every four weeks. Your physician may continue steadily to your lung nodule every year for five years to ensure that it's benign.

Benign nodules also generally have smoother edges and also have a far more even colour throughout and a more natural form than cancerous nodules. Frequently, your physician can check the velocity of growth, style, and other characteristics such as calcification on the upper body X-ray, CT, or Family pet scan. Your physician may order other checks too, particularly if the nodule changes in proportions, form, or appearance; these may be achieved to eliminate the tumour or determine a root reason behind the harmless nodule, they could also help identify any problems. You might have a number of these testing:

- Blood tests.

- Tuberculin epidermis test to check on for TB.

- Positron emission tomography (Family pet) scan.

- Single-photo emission CT (SPECT).

- Magnetic resonance imaging (in rare circumstances).

- Biopsy, cells removal, and exam under a microscope to verify if the tumour is harmless or cancerous.

A biopsy can be carried out utilizing a variety of methods such as aspirating cells through a needle or removing an example of these using bronchoscopy. This process allows your physician to check out your airway through a slim viewing instrument.

Treatment of Benign Lung Nodules and Tumours

Often, your physician may observe a suspicious lung nodule with multiple chest X-rays over many years. However, your physician may suggest a biopsy or removal of a whole nodule in situations like these:

- You are a smoker, and the nodule is large.
- You have symptoms.
- A check suggests the nodule might be cancerous.
- The nodule is continuing to grow.

Surgery can frequently be finished with small incisions and a brief hospital stay. In case your nodule is harmless, you won't need any more treatment except to control any root problems or problems related to the nodule, such as pneumonia or a blockage. If you want invasive surgery to eliminate a tumour, your physician may recommend several exams beforehand, these might include bloodstream lab tests or kidney, liver organ, or pulmonary (lung) function assessments. If needed, surgery may involve one of the methods; the operation depends on the positioning and the kind of your tumour or tumours. The doctor may remove a little bit of tumour, several parts of a lobe, several lobes of the lung, or a whole lung. However, the cosmetic surgeon will remove only a small amount of tissue as you possibly can.

Chapter 7
What's Metastatic Lung Malignancy?

When a tumour develops, it typically forms in a single area or organ of your body. This area is recognized as the leading site. Unlike other cells in the torso, cancer cells can break from the leading site and happen to be other areas of your body.

Tumour cells can move around in your body through the bloodstream or the lymph system. The lymph system comprises of vessels that bring liquids and support the disease fighting capability. When cancer cells happen to be other organs in the torso, it's called *metastasis*. Cancers that metastasize to the lungs is a life-threatening condition that develops when malignancy in another section of the body spreads to the lung. The tumour that evolves at any significant site can develop metastatic tumours; these tumours can grow to the lungs. Main tumours that commonly pass on to the lungs include:

- Bladder cancer.

- Breast cancer.

- Colon cancer.

- Kidney cancer.

- Neuroblastoma.

- Prostate cancer.

- Sarcoma.

- Wilms' tumour

What exactly are the symptoms of metastatic lung tumour?

Metastatic lung cancer doesn't always cause symptoms; when symptoms do develop, they could be difficult to recognize; this is because the symptoms may be just like health conditions besides cancer.

The symptoms of metastatic lung cancer range from:

- A persistent cough.

- Coughing up blood vessels or bloody phlegm.

- Chest pain.

- Shortness of breath.
- Wheezing.
- Weakness.
- Unexpected weight loss.

How does metastatic lung cancers develop?

For malignancy cells to metastasize, they need to proceed through several changes. First, the cells have to break from the leading site and discover ways to enter the bloodstream or lymph system; once they're in the bloodstream or lymph system, the tumour cells must attach themselves to a vessel that allows them to go to a new organ. Regarding metastatic lung cancers, the malignancy cells happen to be the lungs.

When the cells reach the lung, they'll need to improve again to be able to develop in the new location. The cells must have the ability to survive episodes from the disease fighting capability. Many of these changes make metastatic tumour different from principal cancer; this implies that individuals can have two different kinds of cancers.

How is metastatic lung malignancy diagnosed?

Your physician will execute a physical exam and order various diagnostic checks if metastatic cancers are suspected. Your physician will confirm your medical diagnosis by utilizing a diagnostic test, such as:

- *Upper body X-ray*: This test creates complete images of the lung.

- *CT check*: This test produces clear, cross-sectional pictures of the lung.

- *Lung needle biopsy*: Your physician removes a little test of lung tissues for analysis.

- *Bronchoscopy*: Your physician can directly imagine all the buildings that define your respiratory system, like the lungs, with a little camera and light.

How is metastatic lung tumour treated?

The purpose of treatment is to regulate the growth of cancer or even to relieve any observable symptoms (you'll find so many different treatments available). Your unique treatment solution depends on various factors, including:

- Your age.

- Your current health.

- Your health backgrounds.

- Type of principal tumour.

- Located area of the tumour.

- Size of the tumour.

- Quantity of tumours.

Chemotherapy is often used to take care of metastatic cancers to the lungs; this medication therapy helps eliminate cancerous cells in the torso. It's the most well-liked treatment option when the malignancy is more complex and has passed on to other organs in the torso.

In some instances, surgery can also be performed to eliminate the metastatic tumours in the lung. Usually, this is done if someone already experienced their primary tumour removed or if the malignancy has only passed on to limited regions of the lung.

Your doctor could also recommend:

- <u>Radiation</u>: High-energy rays shrinks tumours and destroy cancer cells.

- <u>Laser beam therapy</u>: High-intensity light destroys tumours and tumour cells.

- <u>Stents</u>: Your physician places tiny pipes in the airways to keep them open up.

- <u>Experimental treatments for metastatic cancer are also available</u>: Warmth probes may be used to ruin cancer tumour cells in the lungs. Chemotherapy drugs can also be applied right to the affected section of the lung made up of the metastatic tumour.

What's the long-term perspective for individuals with metastatic lung cancers?

Your long-term outlook depends on the scale and location of most of your tumour. It'll also rely on how much the malignancy has passed on. Certain malignancies that spread to the lungs can be quite treatable with chemotherapy. Primary tumours in the kidney, colon, or bladder that pass on to the lungs may sometimes be removed entirely with surgery.

Generally, metastatic cancer can't be cured; however, treatments can help prolong your daily life and enhance the quality you will ever have.

How can metastatic lung tumour be prevented?

It's tough to avoid metastatic cancers to the lungs. Experts will work on precautionary treatments, but there is nothing common practice yet. One step toward preventing metastatic cancer is the quick and successful treatment of most of your cancer.

Dealing with metastatic lung cancer

It's essential to indeed have a strong support network that will help you with any anxiety and stress you might be feeling. You might consult with a *counsellor or join a cancer support group* where you can discuss your concerns with other people who can relate to what you're going through; ask your physician about organizations locally. *The National Cancer Tumour Institute Trusted Source and American Cancers Culture websites* also offer resources and information on organizations.

Chapter 8

When Lung Malignancy Spreads to the Brain

Lung cancer may spread to the brain in about 40 percent of individuals when metastasis has occurred; metastasis is the medical term used to spell out cancer which includes; spread beyond the original tumour to another, distant body organ system. With lung malignancy, this is known as stage 4 of the condition.

Brain metastases with lung cancer once heralded an unhealthy prognosis, with life span usually being under a year. Conventional treatments for brain metastases, such as chemotherapy are usually ineffective, given that they do not mix the bloodstream brain barrier. Lately, there's been more expect at least some individuals.

Some drugs in the newer treatment categories classified as targeted therapies or immunotherapy can cross this hurdle, and when an individual or just a few brain metastases can be found, local treatment (such as SBRT) of the metastases can, in some instances, lead to long-term control of the condition.

Symptoms of lung tumour with brain metastases

When metastases happen in people who have lung cancers, the other malignancy is not considered a "brain malignancy" but instead "lung tumour metastatic to the brain" or "lung cancers with brain metastases." On the other hand, the word brain cancer is utilized for those tumours which originate in the brain as the principal, rather than supplementary, malignancy. Quite simple, if you were to have a test of the malignancy cells in the brain, they might be cancerous lung cells, not cancerous brain cells.

Sadly, lung malignancies with metastases to the brain have a comparatively poor prognosis, but this is changing for a lot. Unlike many chemotherapy drugs, a few of the newer targeted therapies for lung tumour can penetrate the blood-brain hurdle and can help battle lung tumours that have pass on to the brain. There are also new possibilities for individuals who have just a few metastases to the brain (sometimes thought as *oligometastases*).

The average survival time with brain metastases is usually significantly less than a year, however, when only isolated metastases (oligometastases) are located and can be treated, over 60 percent of individuals may survive for just two years or longer. Furthermore, people who can be treated with some targeted treatments can survive much longer.

When you have lung cancers with brain metastases, your treatment and prognosis may vary, than for someone with the same condition only a couple of years ago. It is critical to learn whatever you can and become your advocate; for example, *a 2018 research found that individuals who are treated with appropriate therapy for ALK-positive lung cancer, the median success rate for people that have stage 4 lung cancer, despite having brain metastases, was 6.8 years.* Regrettably, not everyone identified as having stage 4 non-small cell lung malignancy is tested or offered treatment.

Symptoms

Brain metastases may appear with either small cell lung malignancy or non-small cell lung tumour. Small cell lung tumour is often difficult to diagnose in the first stages and, because of this, may pass on to the brain before an analysis is even made. Non-small cell malignancies can also pass on to the brain but tend to do this later throughout the disease following the main tumour has been found out.

Symptoms may differ based on the kind of lung cancers, and wherein the brain, the metastases occur. As much as another of all people who have secondary brain malignancy will haven't any symptoms whatsoever, and the pass on is available on imaging assessments (like a brain MRI). If indeed they do happen, they typically include:

- Headaches.

- Fatigue.

- Lack of balance.

- Nausea and vomiting.

- Difficulty walking.

- Lack of coordination.

- Speech problems.

- Eyesight changes, including lack of vision or two times vision.

- Peripheral weakness (occurring using one side of your body).

- Memory loss.

- Personality changes.

- Seizures.

Diagnosis

If your physician suspects that your lung cancer has spread to the human brain, she or he will order imaging tests such as computed tomography (CT scan) designed to use X-rays to produce diagnostic images or magnetic resonance imaging (MRI) which does the same with magnetic waves. While an MRI is known as more accurate, it might not be utilized in individuals with certain metallic implants (including non-safe pacemakers).

A different type of imaging tool is *positron emission tomography (PET scan),* which can differentiate between healthy cell metabolism and the ones which appear hyperactive (such as cancer cells). If a suspicious lesion is available, but the analysis is uncertain, a biopsy may be performed to secure a tissue test for evaluation.

Brain Metastases & Leptomeningeal Metastases

Leptomeningeal metastases (leptomeningeal carcinomatosis) tend to be a past due complication of advanced lung tumour, and are being seen additionally as survival rates improve. Unlike brain metastases, leptomeningeal metastases take place when lung cancers cells seed the leptomeninges, the deepest levels of the membranes that surround the brain. Given that they float openly within the cerebrospinal liquid that bathes the brain and spinal cord, they don't need to create large tumours to ensure a way to obtain nutrients.

Symptoms of leptomeningeal metastases often include

multiple neurological symptoms. Treatment can consist of intrathecal chemotherapy (injecting chemotherapy drugs straight into the cerebrospinal liquid) while some targeted drugs, such as some used to take care of EGFR mutations, BRAF mutations, and ALK rearrangements, may enter the vertebral liquid and become useful.

Treatment

The treating brain metastases depend upon lots of factors, including how a lot of the brain is involved as well as your general health. If brain metastases are common, treatment is targeted on managing the symptoms and problems to be able to optimize the standard of living. If there are just a few metastases, local treatment to remove the metastases entirely is often pursued.

Steroids such as *Decadron (dexamethasone)* enable you to control any inflammation of the brain, while anticonvulsive medications (seizure drugs) can decrease the occurrence and intensity of seizures. Other treatments can be divided into general treatments for stage 4 lung malignancy, treatments for wide-spread brain metastases, and localized treatments for oligometastases.

General Treatments

General treatments for cancer include:

- Chemotherapy

Many chemotherapy drugs are inadequate in treating brain metastases because of the existence of the blood-brain barrier, a good network of capillaries which serves to keep toxins (including chemotherapy drugs) from the brain. Chemotherapy may, however, decrease the size of tumours in the lungs and, for that reason, limit their capability to pass on to the brain.

- Targeted Therapy

Targeted drugs for EGFR mutations, ALK rearrangements, ROS rearrangements, as well as others, are sometimes in a position to penetrate the blood-brain barrier. A number of the newer drugs for EGFR mutations, as well as therapies for ALK rearrangements, look very able in dealing with brain metastases. Like chemotherapy, these drugs also control the principal tumour and therefore limit its capability to pass on to the brain.

- Immunotherapy

It's still too early to learn much (the first immunotherapy medication for lung malignancy was approved in 2015); however, the four immunotherapy medications (checkpoint inhibitors) approved for lung tumour show guarantee in their capability to lessen brain metastases. For a lot of, these drugs have resulted in both control of metastases and a "durable response" to the cancers altogether. Relating to a 2018 research released in the *Journal of Clinical Oncology*, checkpoint inhibitors do seem to be effective in dealing with brain metastases; further supported with a 2019 study published in the *Journal of Thoracic Oncology* that found that individuals with non-small cell lung cancer who have been treated with immunotherapy drugs didn't (as could have been expected) have a poorer survival rate if indeed they had brain metastases.

- Entire Brain Radiotherapy

If there are several brain metastases present (malignancy centres vary in defining this, and the quantity may be higher than three to 20), whole-brain radiotherapy has traditionally been recommended. Whole-brain rays may be considered the right choice for individuals who have symptoms related to their brain metastases or who are at risk for problems (like a heart stroke). It may also be used after surgery to lessen further pass on of the tumour, without designed to remedy malignancy, at least 50 percent of individuals going through whole-brain radiotherapy will notice some improvement in symptoms. Common part effects range from memory reduction (especially verbal memory space), pores and skin rash, and exhaustion. Radiation oncologists recommend a medication that seems to reduce cognitive dysfunction related to the treatment.

If whole brain radiotherapy has been recommended for the human brain metastases, talk to your physician about the advantages and drawbacks of the treatment, alternatives available, and medications that may decrease the aspect effects. That is currently a location of controversy in the management of lung cancers; another opinion may be warranted before you begin treatment.

Brain-Metastasis Specific Treatments

Treatments which specifically address brain metastases but made to treat widespread metastases:

- ***Stereotactic Radiotherapy***

This is also called *stereotactic radiosurgery or SBRT*; this is a kind of high-dose radiation directed at a specific section of the brain. Because the rays are targeted, part effects are usually less severe and provide better success rates than whole-brain therapy. This form of radiotherapy is generally reserved for individuals with three or fewer tumours, although many people experienced this treatment for 20 tumours.

- ***Proton Therapy***

Proton therapy can be used in ways much like SBRT and is performed so that they can get rid of the metastases which can be found.

- ***Surgery***

Surgery is utilized less commonly but maybe a choice if there are one or several tumours that are often accessed, and there are no indicators of malignancy elsewhere. Surgery may involve the complete removal of a tumour or incomplete removal to ease symptoms. Whole-brain rays typically come after. Since small-cell tumours are more attentive to radiotherapy only, surgery is more regularly used to eliminate non-small cell malignancies.

- ***Palliative Care***

If the many treatment plans prove ineffective, palliative care enables you to offer alleviation and reduce the stress associated with a terminal diagnosis. This might be the use of *pain medications, physical and occupational therapy, or complementary treatments* to improve comfort and enhance the standard of living.

Brain metastases, thanks to lung tumour can be terrifying, but as frightening as it might be, it is critical to remember that there is no arranged course as it pertains to cancer. It could differ from individual to individual, and the "median" or "average" life expectancies you'll find out about don't always connect with you as a person.

If confronted with brain metastases from lung cancers, use your doctors and family members to help make the most informed choice based on complete and honest disclosure of information. It is beneficial to get another opinion at one of the more prominent National Malignancy Institute-designated malignancy centres which focus on lung tumour. Even if the procedure is the same, your household may feel well informed you are on the right course.

It is essential to allow you to ultimately feel what you are feeling and also to seek support to help navigate this trip. Get in touch with your friends and relations.

There's a very energetic lung cancers community online, and becoming energetic in these organizations will not only bring support from folks who are living an identical trip and "obtain it," but are also a great resource by which to ask questions and find out about the latest improvements in lung malignancy treatment; including those related to the treating brain metastases.

www.ingramcontent.com/pod-product-compliance
Lightning Source LLC
Chambersburg PA
CBHW071114030426
42336CB00013BA/2075